CELIAC DISEASE DIET COOKBOOK:

FOR NEWLY DIAGNOSED

Complete Beginner Procedures On Food Recipes, Guided Meal Plans, And Healthy Lifestyle Tips To Manage, Strive, And Live Well With Celiac Disease

DR. EMMY BROOKS

ABOUT THIS BOOK

The "*CELIAC DISEASE DIET COOKBOOK*" serves as an indispensable guide for individuals navigating the complexities of celiac disease and the essential transition to a gluten-free lifestyle. In its pages, readers embark on a journey of understanding, beginning with a comprehensive exploration of celiac disease itself. From defining the condition to elucidating its common symptoms and signs, the book lays a solid foundation for readers to grasp the intricacies of this autoimmune disorder. Furthermore, it delves into the pivotal role of gluten in exacerbating celiac symptoms, shedding light on hidden sources of gluten and equipping readers with the knowledge needed to make informed dietary choices.

Central to the cookbook's efficacy is its emphasis on the basics of a gluten-free diet. By elucidating which foods to incorporate and avoid, as well as providing guidance on deciphering food labels, the book empowers readers to confidently navigate grocery store aisles and make mindful dietary decisions. Moreover, practical tips for stocking a gluten-free kitchen ensure that readers are well-equipped to embark on their culinary journey with confidence and ease.

The cookbook transcends mere instruction, offering a treasure trove of recipes crafted with both nutrition and flavor in mind. From hearty breakfasts to satisfying dinners and decadent desserts, each recipe is meticulously curated to cater to the diverse palates of individuals adhering to a gluten-free lifestyle. Moreover, with an emphasis on nutrient-rich ingredients and wholesome cooking techniques, the cookbook exemplifies how gluten-free eating can be both nourishing and indulgent.

Beyond the confines of the kitchen, the book extends its guidance to navigating social situations and dining out with celiac disease. By equipping readers with strategies for handling social gatherings and events, the cookbook ensures that individuals can maintain their gluten-free lifestyle without compromising on social experiences.

Ultimately, the "**CELIAC DISEASE DIET COOKBOOK**" stands as a beacon of empowerment, offering not only practical guidance but also encouragement and motivation for embarking on a successful gluten-free journey.

DISCLAIMER

This book's content is solely intended for general informative purposes. About the availability, applicability, correctness, completeness, and trustworthiness of the data or recipes in this book, the author provides no guarantees of any sort, either stated or implied. You bear full responsibility for any reliance you may have on such material.

The advice, diagnosis, or treatment provided by a qualified medical expert is not to be replaced by this cookbook. When in doubt about a medical problem, never hesitate to consult your doctor or another trained healthcare professional. Never ignore medical advice from professionals or put off getting it because of something you've read in this book.

At the time of publishing, the author of this book has taken reasonable steps to guarantee that the information is correct and current. He does not, however, guarantee that the data will be error-free or that it will satisfy any certain performance or quality standards.

Any negative repercussions that may arise from using or applying the material in this book are not the responsibility of the author, publisher, or distributor.

In this book, references or mentions of individuals, products, websites, organizations, or other names are for informational purposes only and do not imply endorsement or affiliation with the author. The author has no control over the nature, content, and availability of referenced or mentioned entities. Any reliance on such information is at the reader's own risk.

The inclusion of any references does not necessarily imply a recommendation or endorse the views expressed within them. The author or publisher shall not be liable for any loss or damage arising out of or in connection with, the use of this book.

INTRODUCTION

UNDERSTANDING CELIAC DISEASE

Understanding Celiac Disease:

For efficient therapy of celiac disease, an autoimmune illness brought on by gluten ingestion, a thorough understanding is necessary. Understanding the fundamentals of this illness is essential to overcoming its obstacles. Fundamentally, celiac disease is an immunological reaction in which eating gluten, a protein present in wheat, barley, and rye, damages the small intestine. This damage then interferes with the body's ability to absorb nutrients, which can lead to a variety of health problems.

Understanding the various symptoms that can appear is crucial to understanding the complexities of celiac disease. In addition to neurological symptoms, anemia, tiredness, and digestive issues are possible in those with celiac disease. Realizing that this illness affects more than just stomach discomfort is essential because it affects many other facets of health. A small intestine biopsy, genetic testing, and blood tests are frequently used in conjunction with diagnosis.

Following a rigorous gluten-free diet is the main treatment for celiac disease once it has been diagnosed. Complications and enduring symptoms may arise from not doing so. It is therefore essential to gain a thorough grasp of the foods that are gluten-containing and to learn how to read ingredient labels. It's also important to be aware of the possibility of cross-contamination because even a small amount of gluten might cause negative effects.

The Significance of a Diet Free of Gluten:

Adopting a gluten-free diet is the cornerstone of managing celiac disease. This dietary change is not just an option—it is required to reduce symptoms, encourage healing, and avert long-term issues. For those who have Celiac disease, gluten—which is found in many grains—acts as an antagonist by triggering an immune response that harms the gut lining.

Going gluten-free is not just about avoiding obvious gluten-containing foods. It demands that people choose their meals carefully, read ingredient labels carefully, and keep an eye out for hidden gluten sources. Knowing the need for this diet means being cautious of less obvious products like sauces, processed foods, and even some drugs that might contain gluten derivatives in addition to avoiding classic sources like bread and pasta.

Living a gluten-free lifestyle does not mean sacrificing nutrient content. It entails switching out gluten-containing grains for gluten-free ones including corn, rice, and quinoa. Finding naturally gluten-free foods such as fruits, vegetables, and proteins is essential to following this diet. In addition, consulting with a trained medical practitioner or nutritionist can offer tailored advice, guaranteeing that dietary requirements are satisfied while adhering to a gluten-free diet.

It may seem intimidating to someone who is not familiar with managing celiac disease to start a gluten-free diet. It is essential to divide the procedure into doable, achievable steps as a result. Every stage should have examples and clear directions, from learning about acceptable and harmful products to becoming an expert at reading labels. People will be able to confidently and easily manage the intricacies of a gluten-free lifestyle with the help of this systematic approach.

CHAPTER ONE

DEFINITION OF CELIAC DISEASE.

Celiac Disease Overview:

Gluten, a protein present in wheat, barley, and rye, can cause the small intestine to become affected by the chronic autoimmune condition celiac disease. In those who have celiac disease, gluten sets off an immunological reaction that damages the lining of the small intestine. The villi, which are tiny projections that resemble fingers and are in charge of absorbing nutrients, become weakened and flattened. This reduces the body's ability to absorb vital nutrients, which can cause several health problems.

It is important to recognize that celiac disease is an autoimmune condition. The immune system incorrectly attacks the body's tissues in response to gluten, unlike food allergies, which involve the immune system's reaction to particular proteins. Untreated celiac disease can have long-term effects that include infertility, osteoporosis, malnourishment, and a higher chance of developing other autoimmune disorders.

A small intestine sample is frequently used in conjunction with clinical assessment and blood tests that measure certain antibodies to confirm the diagnosis of celiac disease. Since the only effective therapy is to follow a rigorous gluten-free diet for the rest of one's life, diagnosis is crucial.

Typical Signs and Symptoms:

A wide range of symptoms, which can differ greatly between people, are indicative of celiac disease. Gastrointestinal problems, such as diarrhea, bloating, abdominal pain, and weight loss, are some typical symptoms. Nevertheless, symptoms other than gastrointestinal issues can also be present with celiac disease.

Anemia, exhaustion, and inexplicable weight loss are common symptoms when the damaged small intestine fails to absorb vital nutrients. Dermatitis herpetiformis is one type of skin rash that has been linked to celiac disease. Neural symptoms such as headaches, balance issues, and mood abnormalities could also be present.

Crucially, a lot of people with celiac disease could not show any symptoms at all, which makes diagnosis difficult. It's critical to identify both the prevalent and less obvious symptoms as a result. For an accurate assessment and diagnosis, speaking with a medical expert is crucial if celiac disease is suspected.

A newcomer to celiac disease must comprehend the wide variety of symptoms. People can better understand the complex nature of the illness and seek the right medical advice if they are aware of the symptoms, which go beyond gastrointestinal problems.

CHAPTER TWO

GLUTEN'S IMPACT ON CELIAC DISEASE
Knowing Gluten and How It Affects Those with Celiac Disease

A protein compound called gluten is present in wheat, barley, rye, and their derivatives. It is essential to the structure and texture of a variety of dietary items. But for those who have celiac disease, a chronic autoimmune illness, eating gluten causes the body to react negatively, which damages the small intestine and causes inflammation. For people hoping to effectively manage their celiac disease, understanding the mechanism underlying gluten's effects is essential.

First off, gliadin and glutenin are the two primary protein groups that makeup gluten. Gliadin emerges as a primary cause in celiac disease patients. When a person with celiac disease consumes gluten, their immune system attacks the gluten, harming the villi, which are tiny projections that resemble fingers that line the small intestine and are essential for absorbing nutrients. Damage of this kind can result in malabsorption of vital nutrients, which can cause a variety of symptoms, such as weariness and nutritional shortages in addition to gastrointestinal problems.

A newcomer to celiac disease must have a basic understanding of how gluten affects immune responses. Understanding that it's an autoimmune disease rather than just an intolerance can change how seriously gluten avoidance needs to be taken.

Now, let's dive into doable actions that will enable beginners to recognize and steer clear of hidden gluten sources, which are a crucial part of controlling celiac disease.

Finding Gluten's Hidden Sources:

1. Learning about gluten-containing grains: Getting acquainted with gluten-containing grains is the first step. The main culprits are wheat,

barley, and rye, but derivatives like bulgur, farina, and spelled could also be dangerous.

A beginner should read ingredient lists very carefully and become comfortable identifying these grains in different combinations.

2. Detailed label reading: Beginners need to form the habit of carefully reading food labels. Unexpected locations to find gluten include sauces, condiments, and processed foods. Gluten may be present in ingredients such as hydrolyzed vegetable protein, malt extract, and modified food starch. Being watchful and asking questions about unfamiliar phrases on labels are examples of practical advice.

3. Recognizing the hazards of cross-contamination: Cross-contamination is a common hazard that occurs when gluten-free and gluten-containing meals come into contact. To avoid unintentional exposure, novices require explicit instructions on safe food preparation techniques that emphasize the value of separate utensils,

cooking surfaces, and even specialized gluten-free cooking facilities.

4. Making use of gluten-free substitutes: Adopting a gluten-free diet doesn't have to mean giving up flavor and diversity. Beginners can experiment with a variety of gluten-free substitutes, including almond flour, quinoa, and rice flour. Giving beginners helpful tips on how to cook with these substitutions regularly can enable them to produce delicious, gluten-free meals.

5. Managing difficulties when eating out: For people who are new to having celiac disease, eating out might be frightening. A flawless dining experience depends on advising them on how to tell restaurant employees about their dietary requirements, look for gluten-free menu items, and be wary of possible cross-contamination in restaurant kitchens.

Therefore, Armed with this information, beginners can then confidently and satisfactorily make the transition to a gluten-free living by navigating the challenging process of finding and avoiding hidden sources of gluten with practical actions.

CHAPTER THREE

FUNDAMENTALS OF A DIET FREE OF GLUTEN

Foods to Take and Leave Out

For those with celiac disease, a gluten-free diet is essential since gluten can cause negative reactions in their bodies. Knowing which items to include and which to completely avoid is crucial for effectively navigating this nutritional journey.

Foods to Add:

1. **Naturally Gluten-Free Grains:** Include grains in your diet, like millet, rice, quinoa, and maize. These grains can be adaptable additions to a variety of recipes and are naturally free of gluten.

2. Gluten-Free Flour: Instead of using regular wheat flour in your recipes, try using alternative flours like almond, coconut, or chickpea flour. These substitutes give you a gluten-free choice while also enhancing your food with interesting tastes and textures.

3. Fresh Vegetables and Fruits: Savor a rainbow of vibrant fresh vegetables and fruits. These nutrient-dense options are safe because they naturally don't contain gluten and also support a well-balanced diet.

4. Protein Sources: Emphasize lean meats, eggs, chicken, and fish as gluten-free protein sources. Tofu, beans, and legumes are great plant-based substitutes that may vary the protein in your meals.

5. Dairy and Dairy Alternatives: By nature, most dairy products don't contain gluten. But always be on the lookout for flavorings or chemicals that can contain gluten. Additionally, look into non-dairy options like coconut yogurt or almond milk.

6. Nuts and Seeds: Vary your diet to include a range of nuts and seeds. They add a delightful crunch to your meals or snacks in addition to providing healthy fats and proteins.

Foods to Steer Clear of:

1. Products Made With Wheat: Avoid anything made with wheat, such as baked products, spaghetti, and bread. Check the market for gluten-free substitutes or look into recipes that call for gluten-free flour.

2. Barley and Rye: Steer clear of products that include barley or rye. This includes several processed meals that might contain these grains, as well as some beers and malt vinegar.

3. Processed Foods: Watch out for hidden gluten in processed foods, as they frequently contain it. Look for substances like hydrolyzed wheat protein, modified food starch, and malt extract on labels.

4. Cross-Contaminated Foods: Be cautious when consuming food from other people, particularly in communal kitchen areas or when dining out. To avoid any gluten residue, make sure that all cooking surfaces, cutting boards, and utensils are well-cleaned.

5. Pre-Packaged Sauces and Dressings: As a thickening agent, gluten may be included in several pre-packaged sauces and dressings. To find gluten-free options, choose handmade versions or carefully read labels.

Comprehending and putting these recommendations into practice will lay the groundwork for a successful gluten-free diet, enabling people with celiac disease to eat a wide variety of healthful foods without sacrificing flavor.

Effectively Reading Food Labels

For anyone on a gluten-free diet, being able to read food labels well is essential since it can reveal hidden gluten sources in a variety of items. The grocery store aisles can seem intimidating at first, but anyone can learn to identify gluten-free choices by following a methodical process.

Step 1: Recognize Ingredients Contains Gluten

Get acquainted with substances that indicate gluten content. Rye, wheat, barley, and their derivatives are common offenders.

Watch out for less obvious sources that may contain gluten, such as modified food starch, hydrolyzed wheat protein, and malt flavoring.

Step 2: Seek Certification for Gluten-Free Products

Nowadays, a lot of food products have gluten-free certification, which verifies that they adhere to stringent gluten-free guidelines. Seek out labels or symbols from reliable organizations that certify products as gluten-free, as they assure that the product has been tested and complies with gluten-free standards.

Step 3: Carefully Examine Allergen Data

Allergen information on food labels frequently lists common allergies, such as wheat. You can use this area as a quick reference to find out if a product contains gluten. But be on the lookout—gluten might not always be specifically indicated.

Step 4: Use Processed Foods Cautiously

Foods that have been processed may contain hidden gluten. Read labels on packaged snacks, sauces, and prepared foods carefully. Watch out for phrases like "natural flavors" or "spices," as these can occasionally hide products that contain gluten.

Step 5: Utilize Resources and Apps without Gluten

Make the most of technology by using internet resources and apps that are gluten-free. You may use certain applications to quickly ascertain whether a product is gluten-free by scanning its barcode. Furthermore, forums and websites devoted to gluten-free living can offer insightful advice and product recommendations.

Step 6: Take Cross-Contamination into Consideration

It is important to take into account the possibility of cross-contamination even with gluten-free products. Pay attention to labels that state that no cross-contamination with gluten-containing items has occurred or that they are manufactured using gluten-free methods.

With these guidelines in hand and a critical eye on product labels, those following a gluten-free diet may make educated decisions with confidence, guaranteeing that their meals meet their dietary needs. With practice, this ability becomes automatic, enabling people to easily sustain a gluten-free lifestyle.

CHAPTER FOUR

PUTTING TOGETHER A GLUTEN-FREE KITCHEN

Crucial Items for a Gluten-Free Pantry:

Purchasing a range of flour substitutes is one of the first steps towards equipping your gluten-free kitchen. Next, get baking essentials. Use gluten-free alternatives such as tapioca, rice, almond, and coconut flour in place of regular wheat flour. Many recipes can employ these substitutes in a one-to-one ratio, facilitating a seamless changeover. Furthermore, think about stocking your cupboard with xanthan gum, a popular gluten alternative that gives gluten-free baked goods flexibility.

Grain and Cereal Variety: Add a variety of gluten-free grains and cereals to your gluten-free cupboard. Excellent options include quinoa, brown rice, millet, and gluten-free oats. These grains offer a range of textures and aromas, making them useful as meal foundations.

Check the label to make sure the grains you buy are gluten-free at all times because processing might lead to cross-contamination.

Gluten-Free Pasta & Noodles: Bid adieu to conventional pasta made from wheat and hello to gluten-free substitutes. Choose noodles manufactured from other grains, such as quinoa or chickpea, or rice or corn pasta. These options are easily substituted for your favorite pasta meals and can be found in most grocery stores.

Condiments and Sauces: It's important to select gluten-free options because many condiments and sauces have hidden gluten in them. Keep tamari, Worcestershire sauce, and gluten-free soy sauce stocked in your kitchen. Additionally, make sure there are no gluten-containing substances on the labels of salad dressings, ketchup, and mustard.

Legumes and tinned foods: To increase the nutritious content of your meals, stock your pantry with a range of legumes and tinned foods. Naturally gluten-free, beans, lentils, and chickpeas can be utilized in a wide variety of dishes.

Verify the gluten-free status of canned soups and broths by reading the labels, as some may have thickeners made of wheat.

Snack Options: To have quick and easy options, keep a variety of gluten-free snacks on hand. Nuts, popcorn, rice cakes, and gluten-free crackers are all great options. When it comes to flavored snacks, exercise caution and always check the labels to be sure they're gluten-free.

Milk and Dairy Substitutes: Although the majority of dairy products are inherently gluten-free, it's important to be aware of flavored or processed varieties that can include gluten additions. Make sure the dairy substitutes you choose—like almond or coconut milk—are labeled as gluten-free.

Sweeteners and Baking Additives: Use gluten-free honey, maple syrup, or agave nectar in place of conventional sweeteners. Baking soda and flourless baking powder are also essential additions to your pantry.

These ingredients guarantee that your baked items rise correctly without requiring gluten.

Organizing a Kitchen That's Celiac-Friendly: Some Advice

Establish Gluten-Free Zones: To reduce the possibility of cross-contamination, set aside specific areas in your kitchen for gluten-free products. Store gluten-free flour, snacks, and utensils in different drawers, shelves, or containers. This group promotes safer cooking conditions and assists in preventing inadvertent mixing.

Labeling and Organizing: Make sure your gluten-free products have labels that are easy to read and crystal clear. Labeling jars, storage bags, and containers can help you avoid confusion and give immediate visual confirmation that the products you have are gluten-free. To expedite your cooking process, divide your pantry into areas designated for cereals, canned foods, and baking supplies.

Separate Cooking Utensils and Appliances: Set aside particular cooking utensils and appliances for gluten-free cooking to prevent cross-contamination when preparing food. Keep toaster ovens, colanders, and cutting boards apart for gluten-free foods. This lessens the possibility of gluten crumbs finding their way into gluten-free meals.

Teach Your Family and Roommates: Make sure that everyone in your home is aware of the significance of keeping your home gluten-free. Teach your family and roommates the dangers of cross-contamination and the importance of keeping gluten-containing and gluten-free equipment and cooking areas apart.

Check Ingredients and Labels Frequently: Pay close attention to label reading, even for items you've already bought. Manufacturers may alter ingredients or processing techniques, so it's important to periodically check labels to keep informed and make sure your pantry stays gluten-free.

Plan and Prepare Gluten-Free Meals: By organizing and preparing gluten-free meals in advance, you may make becoming gluten-free easier. During hectic days, you can save time by preparing gluten-free essentials like quinoa, rice, and gluten-free pasta in bulk. Making a meal plan helps you resist the need to eat gluten-containing convenience items.

Look for Gluten-Free Certification: Select gluten-free certified items whenever possible. Many manufacturers choose to go through the voluntary gluten-free certification processes, giving those who have celiac disease an additional level of security. To make sure packaged goods adhere to strict gluten-free guidelines, look for credible gluten-free labels.

You may safely supply your gluten-free kitchen and arrange it to reduce the chance of cross-contamination, providing a safe and comfortable cooking environment for persons with celiac disease, by putting these doable measures and advice into practice.

CHAPTER FIVE

COOKING WITH GLUTEN-FREE FLOURS

An Overview of Alternatives to Gluten-Free Flour

Knowing the many gluten-free flour options is essential for effective and pleasurable cooking when starting a Celiac Disease Diet. For those with celiac disease, gluten—a protein present in wheat, barley, and rye—must be avoided. Thank goodness, there are several of gluten-free flours out now, each with special qualities to suit different cooking requirements.

Rice flour is a common option because of its many uses. White rice flour has a gentler taste and is best used for delicate cakes and cookies, while brown rice flour, with its nutty flavor, is great for bread and pastries. Almond flour is a tasty and nutrient-dense choice that gives baked items a rich, nutty taste. It is prepared from ground almonds. Because coconut flour is made from dried coconut meat, it absorbs a lot of moisture and gives a delicate coconut flavor to dishes.

Chickpea flour has a somewhat nutty flavor and a solid texture, making it a great option for anyone looking to increase their protein intake. Contrary to its name, buckwheat flour is gluten-free and has a unique earthy flavor that makes it perfect for soba noodles and pancakes. Made from quinoa seeds, quinoa flour gives baked foods a nutty flavor and is a full protein source. Your Celiac Disease Diet can be varied and satisfying by experimenting with different gluten-free flours.

Useful Advice for Succeeding with Gluten-Free Baking

For those who have never baked gluten-free, navigating the world of baking might be frightening, but with a few helpful pointers, it can be a fun and profitable endeavor. Priority one should be given to being acquainted with the unique characteristics of the gluten-free flour you are using. Every flour has a unique behavior that impacts flavor, texture, and moisture absorption. Gaining the appropriate outcomes from your recipes requires an understanding of these subtleties.

Binding agents play an important role in baking that is free of gluten. Because there is no gluten, adding binders such as guar gum or xanthan gum is necessary to keep the crumbles from disintegrating. Small amounts of these, usually 1/4 to 1/2 teaspoon per cup of gluten-free flour, can be added to recipes. Since eggs are essential for binding, a recipe's egg content may need to be changed for the best consistency.

Moisture management is another essential component. Compared to regular flours, gluten-free flours frequently absorb more liquid, which produces dry and crumbly results. Increase the amount of liquid—water, milk, or other liquids—in your recipes to combat this. Furthermore, adding wet ingredients to your gluten-free baked products, such as yogurt, applesauce, or mashed fruit, improves their overall texture and moisture content.

Both baking time and temperature are important. Goods free of gluten might need to bake at lower temperatures for longer periods. Make sure your products are cooked through by using the toothpick test and keeping a careful check on them. The secret to perfecting gluten-free baking is perseverance and experimenting, so don't be afraid to modify and improve your strategy in light of your unique tastes and experiences.

CHAPTER SIX

GLUTEN-FREE, NUTRIENT-RICH INGREDIENTS
Including Nutritious and Wholesome Ingredients in Gluten-Free Meals:

When starting a gluten-free diet, it's important to concentrate on adding healthful and nourishing ingredients to make sure that your meals are high in vital nutrients and suitable for those with celiac disease. The vitamins, minerals, and fiber that may be missing from a gluten-free diet can be obtained with a well-balanced diet that excludes gluten-containing grains.

1. Select entire, Unprocessed Foods: When creating your gluten-free meals, choose entire, unprocessed foods as the main ingredient. Nuts, seeds, legumes, fresh produce, and lean meats are all great options. These organic, natural foods assist you in diversifying your nutrient intake in addition to improving general health.

2. Examine Gluten-Free Grains: Although conventional grains like rye, barley, and wheat are forbidden, there are many gluten-free substitutes out today. Because of their adaptability, brown rice, buckwheat, millet, and quinoa can be substituted in a variety of recipes. Trying out various gluten-free grains will spice up your dishes and keep them engaging.

3. Add Nutrient-Dense Gluten-Free Flours: Instead of using regular wheat flour, switch to nutrient-dense gluten-free flour. Great substitutes include almond flour, coconut flour, chickpea flour, and sorghum flour. These flours provide your recipes with distinctive aromas and textures in addition to acting as a gluten-free foundation.

4. Put Lean Proteins First: Make sure that enough lean proteins—like those found in fish, chicken, tofu, lentils, and eggs—are included in your gluten-free meals. A range of protein sources can enhance the taste and nutritional value of your meals. Proteins are necessary for the growth of muscle.

5. Accept Dairy and Dairy replacements: To get additional calcium and vitamin D, you can consume dairy or dairy replacements such as soy milk, almond milk, or coconut milk. These dairy alternatives also have a creamy texture, which makes your gluten-free recipes look better overall.

6. Include Healthy Fats: Don't be afraid to include healthy fats in your gluten-free cooking. Nuts, seeds, avocado, and olive oil are good sources of good fats that promote well-being and fullness.

7. Mindful Seasoning with Herbs and Spices: Use a range of herbs and spices to enhance the flavor of your gluten-free recipes. Herbs and spices not only impart flavor without requiring gluten-containing seasonings, but many of them have additional health advantages.

Emphasizing Superfoods Free of Gluten:

Some superfoods are more notable than others when it comes to gluten-free cuisine because of their superior nutritional profiles and recipe adaptability. By incorporating these superfoods into your celiac disease diet, you may add new and intriguing flavors to your cooking arsenal while also ensuring a well-rounded nutrient intake.

1. Quinoa: Known as a complete protein, quinoa is a superfood that is free of gluten and contains all of the essential amino acids. With its fluffy texture and nutty flavor, it works well as a side dish or as a basis for salads.

2. Chia Seeds: Rich in fiber, antioxidants, and omega-3 fatty acids, chia seeds are a nutritional powerhouse. They can be added to smoothies, used to make gluten-free puddings, or sprinkled over yogurt to offer an extra nutritional boost.

3. Sweet potatoes are a versatile, gluten-free superfood that is high in vitamins, minerals, and fiber. For extra nutritious benefits, roast them as fries, mash them as a side dish, or add them to soups and stews.

4. Berries: In addition to being delicious, berries like blueberries, strawberries, and raspberries are also a great source of fiber, vitamins, and antioxidants. Enjoy them as a stand-alone snack or mix them into yogurt or gluten-free cereals.

5. Salmon: Omega-3 fatty acids, which are vital for heart health, are abundant in fatty fish like salmon. Salmon makes a delicious and gluten-free main meal whether grilled or baked.

6. Kale: A nutrient-dense leafy green that is high in fiber and packed with vitamins A, C, and K. Increase the nutritious value of your gluten-free meals by adding it to salads, smoothies, or sautéed vegetables as a side dish.

7. Legumes: Packed with fiber and protein, beans and lentils are also free of gluten. Add them to salads, stews, or soups for a filling and healthy gluten-free dinner.

These healthy, nutrient-dense ingredients can be combined with gluten-free superfoods to produce a wide variety of tasty meals that meet the dietary requirements of people with celiac disease. Trying different combinations of these items can not only please your palate but also improve your general health.

CHAPTER EIGHT

EASY AND TASTY BREAKFAST RECIPES WITHOUT GLUTEN

Easy and gluten-free breakfast options:

If you have celiac disease, being gluten-free doesn't have to mean compromising taste or diversity, especially when it comes to breakfast, which is the most crucial meal of the day. You can enjoy a wide variety of easy, gluten-free morning meals that will fill you up and give you energy with a little bit of creativity and tweaking.

A delicious and easy choice is a yogurt parfait made without gluten. Start by choosing a yogurt that has been certified gluten-free and making sure it doesn't have any unidentified gluten-containing thickeners or chemicals. Serve it with your preferred gluten-free granola, or even better, whip up some yourself by mixing nuts, seeds, and gluten-free oats.

Arrange the granola and yogurt in a glass or bowl, then garnish with sliced or fresh fruit for a touch of sweetness. This tasty parfait has a pleasing appearance and is easy to put together. It has a good amount of protein, fiber, and vitamins.

Oatmeal without gluten is a traditional option for people who want a warm start to the day. Select oats that have been verified gluten-free to prevent any possible cross-contamination. Make the oats with your preferred nondairy milk or water, and use natural sweeteners like honey or maple syrup to provide a hint of sweetness. To improve the flavor, add some fresh fruit, nuts, or seeds. For added convenience for newcomers, try utilizing instant gluten-free oatmeal packets. This choice guarantees a safe gluten-free experience while enabling a rapid and hassle-free preparation.

A smoothie bowl without gluten is an additional quick and healthy breakfast option. Start by choosing a gluten-free protein powder and making sure it doesn't contain any gluten-containing ingredients.

Blend the protein powder with your preferred dairy-free milk or yogurt along with frozen fruits, like berries or bananas. Transfer the smoothie into a bowl and garnish with sliced fruits, nuts, seeds, and gluten-free granola for some extra taste and texture. This colorful and adaptable meal gives you a nutrient-rich start to the day while also satisfying your taste buds.

Easy and delectable breakfast options:

Having tasty and quick gluten-free breakfast options on hand can make all the difference when time is important. A quick and pleasant option might be a gluten-free breakfast burrito. To begin with, select gluten-free tortillas, which are widely accessible in most supermarkets. For a vegan option, use tofu or scrambled eggs, then sauté your favorite veggies, such as spinach, onions, and bell peppers. Top with avocado slices, cheese, and a dab of spicy sauce or gluten-free salsa. Roll the contents into the tortilla to make a tasty, on-the-go breakfast that is portable and flavorful.

A quick alternative might be a stack of gluten-free banana pancakes. Mash bananas, gluten-free flour, baking powder, and a small amount of vanilla essence to make a basic batter. Small pancakes should be cooked till golden brown on a hot griddle. Garnish the pancakes with chopped nuts, fresh berries, and a drizzle of maple syrup. You don't need to make complicated preparations to enjoy a delicious breakfast with this fuss-free pancake recipe.

A wonderful option for individuals who want a heartier start to the day is a gluten-free breakfast sandwich. Start by toasting gluten-free bread or using an English muffin that has already been prepared. For a plant-based substitute, cook some bacon or sausage without gluten, scramble some eggs, or make some tofu scramble. Top the sandwich with your favorite condiments, including avocado, mayonnaise, or mustard. This filling and flavorful breakfast alternative is perfect for hectic mornings because it can be made in a matter of minutes.

Therefore, these easy and quick breakfast alternatives free of gluten satisfy the requirements of people following a celiac disease diet and provide a satisfying start to the day. These recipes offer a variety of options for a gluten-free diet, whether you choose a yogurt parfait, oatmeal, smoothie bowl, breakfast burrito, banana pancake stack, or breakfast sandwich. Even beginners can confidently cook these delectable breakfasts, which set the tone for a fulfilling and nourishing day ahead with simple-to-follow instructions and easily accessible materials.

CHAPTER EIGHT

WHOLESOME LUNCHES FOR A GLUTEN-FREE LIFESTYLE

Nutrient-Packed Gluten-Free Lunch Ideas:

If you have celiac disease, becoming gluten-free doesn't have to mean compromising on taste or nutrition. There are, in fact, a plethora of nutrient-dense selections that will not only satisfy your palate but also meet your nutritional requirements. Come along as we discuss some healthy, nutrient-dense, and simple gluten-free lunch alternatives.

A salad with quinoa and vegetables is a great option. Grain devoid of gluten, quinoa is a nutritious powerhouse with an extensive protein profile and an abundance of vitamins and minerals. To make this salad, cook the quinoa following the directions on the package and combine it with a variety of vibrant, fresh veggies, such as bell peppers, cucumbers, cherry tomatoes, and red onions.

Add a handful of chopped herbs, like parsley or cilantro, to enhance the flavor. Drizzle with a tangy vinaigrette composed of olive oil, balsamic vinegar, Dijon mustard, and a tiny bit of honey— all gluten-free ingredients. This recipe offers a delightful crunch along with a healthful and well-balanced dinner.

Stuffed bell peppers, which are free of gluten, are a more substantial choice. These tasty and highly protein-dense peppers are stuffed with quinoa, black beans, mixed vegetables, and minced turkey or chicken. For a taste explosion, add gluten-free herbs and spices to the filling, such as oregano, cumin, and paprika. Once the peppers are soft, you'll have a wholesome dinner that's convenient to reheat all week long.

A creative and nutrient-dense alternative is a stir-fried tofu and vegetables that are free of gluten. Made from soybeans, tofu is a great source of protein and is naturally gluten-free. A variety of vibrant veggies, including bell peppers, carrots, snap peas, and broccoli, can be sautéed in gluten-free soy or tamari sauce. After adding the cubed tofu, stir-fry everything until it's well-cooked. For a filling and nutritious lunch that's high in taste and nutrients, serve over rice noodles or gluten-free rice.

These creative and tasty gluten-free lunch ideas highlight the variety of tasty options available while still meeting the dietary requirements of those who suffer from celiac disease. Trying out different gluten-free grains, meats, and veggies can keep your meals interesting, fulfilling, and—most importantly—nutrient-dense.

Lunch Ideas That Are Handsome and Convenient for People with Celiac Disease:

Planning meals is very important when you have celiac disease, especially for lunches, which must be easy to carry and convenient. Having portable, gluten-free lunch options is crucial, whether you're heading to work, school, or other everyday activities. Let's look at some doable and hassle-free suggestions to help you lead a more joyful and manageable gluten-free existence.

The wrap provides a flexible choice that is free of gluten. Choose a wrap or tortilla without gluten that is manufactured with rice, maize, or chickpea flour instead of regular flour. Top it with a variety of gluten-free meats, such as turkey, tofu, or grilled chicken, then top it with your preferred gluten-free condiments, fresh veggies, and greens. For a tidy and portable lunch on the run, roll it tightly and cover it with aluminum foil or parchment paper.

Consider making salads in mason jars that are gluten-free as a quick and convenient option. Organizing your components into layers will guarantee that your salad stays crisp and fresh until it's time to eat. Start with a gluten-free dressing at the bottom, then add protein, robust veggies, and lush greens on the top. To enjoy your gluten-free salad on the go, just shake the jar to evenly distribute the dressing when it's time to eat.

One of the best options for a portable and warm lunch is soup. Make a big pot of gluten-free soup, like a thick chicken or vegetable soup, and transfer it into separate, airtight jars. When needed, reheat, and you'll have a satisfying and portable gluten-free lunch alternative that you can take with you wherever.

Another wise move is to include gluten-free grains in your carry-along lunches. You may cook quinoa, rice, and gluten-free pasta ahead of time and serve them with different types of veggies and proteins. These lunch ideas are tasty and convenient to pack for travel, requiring little preparation on your hectic days. Just make sure to store them in sealed containers.

With the help of these easy and transportable gluten-free lunch options, people with celiac disease can continue to follow their dietary restrictions and yet enjoy tasty, hassle-free meals. The hurdles of living a gluten-free lifestyle can be easily navigated, even when traveling, with a little preparation and ingenuity.

CHAPTER NINE

DELIGHTFUL DINNERS WITHOUT GLUTEN

Dinner Recipes: Delicious Gluten-Free Recipes

Navigating a gluten-free diet can feel daunting, especially when it comes to dinner time. But fear not, because this section is packed with delicious and satisfying dinner recipes that are completely gluten-free. Whether you're cooking for yourself, your family, or entertaining guests, these recipes will surely impress without compromising on flavor or texture.

Let's break it down step by step to make it easy for novices to follow along and create scrumptious gluten-free dinners with confidence.

Step 1: Choose Your Base Ingredients

Before diving into the recipes, it's essential to stock up on gluten-free staples for your kitchen. Make sure to have plenty of gluten-free grains like rice, quinoa, and gluten-free pasta on hand. Other pantry essentials include gluten-free flour blends, breadcrumbs, and sauces labeled as gluten-free. By having these basics at your disposal, you'll be ready to tackle any recipe with ease.

Step 2: Explore Flavorful Proteins

Next, let's consider the protein options for your gluten-free dinners. Whether you prefer poultry, seafood, tofu, or legumes, there are plenty of delicious options to choose from. Think about incorporating lean proteins like chicken breast, turkey, or fish into your meals for a healthy boost. Additionally, experiment with plant-based proteins like chickpeas, lentils, or quinoa for hearty and nutritious dinner options.

Step 3: Get Creative with Vegetables

Vegetables are the cornerstone of any nutritious meal, and they play a crucial role in gluten-free cooking. Embrace a rainbow of colors by including a variety of fresh, frozen, or canned vegetables in your recipes.

From leafy greens and cruciferous veggies to vibrant bell peppers and sweet potatoes, there's no shortage of options to add flavor, texture, and nutrients to your gluten-free dinners.

Step 4: Elevate with Herbs and Spices

Herbs and spices are the secret weapons that can elevate any dish from ordinary to extraordinary. Experiment with different flavor profiles by incorporating a variety of herbs like basil, cilantro, and parsley, along with aromatic spices such as cumin, paprika, and garlic powder. These flavorful additions will enhance the taste of your gluten-free dinners and make them truly unforgettable.

Step 5: Try One-Pot Wonders

One-pot dinners are a game-changer for busy weeknights when you want a delicious meal without the hassle of multiple pots and pans. Explore recipes like gluten-free stir-fries, casseroles, and sheet pan dinners that require minimal cleanup and maximum flavor. With just one pot or pan, you can create a wholesome and satisfying meal that the whole family will love.

Step 6: Embrace Simple Dinner Ideas

Sometimes, the simplest dinners are the most satisfying. Keep things easy and stress-free by incorporating simple dinner ideas into your gluten-free meal rotation. From grilled chicken with roasted vegetables to quinoa salad with avocado and black beans, there are endless possibilities for quick and tasty gluten-free dinners that require minimal effort but deliver maximum satisfaction.

By following these practical steps and exploring the diverse range of dinner recipes provided, novices can confidently navigate the world of gluten-free cooking and enjoy delightful dinners without any confusion.

One-Pot Dinners & Simple Dinner Ideas:

When it comes to preparing dinner, simplicity and convenience are key, especially for those following a gluten-free diet. That's where one-pot dinners and simple dinner ideas come into play, offering delicious and hassle-free meals that require minimal cleanup and preparation time. Whether you're a novice cook or a seasoned chef, these practical and straightforward recipes are sure to become staples in your gluten-free meal repertoire.

Step 1: Choose Your One-Pot Wonder

The beauty of one-pot dinners lies in their simplicity and versatility. Start by selecting a recipe that appeals to your taste preferences and dietary needs. From hearty soups and stews to flavorful pasta dishes and grain bowls, there's no shortage of options to explore. Consider ingredients that cook well together in a single pot or pan, making cleanup a breeze and saving you valuable time in the kitchen.

Step 2: Prep Your Ingredients

Once you've chosen your one-pot wonder, it's time to gather and prepare your ingredients. Chop vegetables, measure out spices, and portion protein sources to streamline the cooking process. Prepping ingredients ahead of time not only saves time but also ensures that everything is ready to go when it's time to start cooking. Plus, it allows for easy customization based on personal preferences and dietary restrictions.

Step 3: Follow the Recipe Instructions

Now it's time to put your one-pot dinner together following the recipe instructions provided. Start by heating oil or butter in a large pot or skillet, then sauté aromatics like onions, garlic, and spices to build flavor. Add your protein source and cook until browned, then incorporate vegetables, grains, or pasta along with any liquids like broth or sauce. Cover and simmer until everything is cooked through and flavors have melded together.

Step 4: Serve and Enjoy

Once your one-pot dinner is ready, it's time to serve and enjoy! Divide the meal into individual portions and garnish with fresh herbs, grated cheese, or a squeeze of lemon juice for added flavor. Serve alongside gluten-free bread, crackers, or a simple side salad for a complete and satisfying meal. Don't forget to savor each bite and appreciate the simplicity and convenience of one-pot cooking.

Step 5: Clean Up: The best part about one-pot dinners is the minimal cleanup required. Simply wash the pot or pan used for cooking, along with any utensils and cutting boards, and your kitchen will be sparkling clean in no time. This hassle-free cleanup process makes one-pot dinners ideal for busy weeknights when you'd rather spend time relaxing with loved ones than scrubbing pots and pans.

By following these practical steps and embracing the simplicity of one-pot dinners and simple dinner ideas, novices can confidently whip up delicious gluten-free meals with ease and enjoyment. Whether you're cooking for yourself, your family, or entertaining guests, these recipes are sure to delight and satisfy without any confusion.

More Delicious Gluten-Free Dinner Recipes

1. Quinoa and Vegetable Stir-Fry:

Preparation Tips:

Begin by rinsing and cooking quinoa according to package instructions. Use a non-stick skillet or wok for the stir-fry to minimize the need for excessive oil. Chop your favorite gluten-free vegetables such as bell peppers, broccoli, and carrots into bite-sized pieces. Have gluten-free soy sauce or tamari on hand for added flavor. Prepping ingredients ahead will streamline the cooking process.

Recipe:

In a preheated skillet, sauté chopped garlic and ginger in a small amount of oil.

Add sliced chicken or tofu and cook until browned.

Toss in the chopped vegetables and stir-fry until they are crisp-tender.

Incorporate cooked quinoa into the mix and pour in gluten-free soy sauce or tamari.

Mix everything together until thoroughly mixed and hot.

Garnish with chopped green onions and sesame seeds before serving.

2. Baked Lemon Herb Salmon with Quinoa Pilaf:

Preparation Tips:

Preheat your oven for efficient baking. Choose a gluten-free herb seasoning blend or prepare a mix of your favorite herbs such as thyme, rosemary, and parsley. Ensure the salmon fillets are fresh and properly thawed if frozen. Rinse and cook quinoa, adding a squeeze of lemon juice for a refreshing flavor.

Recipe:

Place salmon fillets on a baking sheet lined with parchment paper.

Drizzle olive oil over the salmon and sprinkle the herb seasoning generously.

Bake in the preheated oven until the salmon is cooked through and flakes easily.

In a separate pot, sauté onions and garlic in olive oil, then add quinoa.

Pour in gluten-free chicken or vegetable broth and let it simmer until the quinoa is cooked.

Fluff the quinoa with a fork and stir in freshly chopped parsley and a squeeze of lemon juice.

Serve the baked lemon herb salmon on a bed of quinoa pilaf.

3. Gluten-Free Margherita Pizza with Cauliflower Crust:

Preparation Tips:

Purchase or make gluten-free cauliflower pizza crust in advance. Choose fresh and ripe tomatoes for the sauce and fresh mozzarella for a classic Margherita flavor. Keep a selection of fresh basil leaves for garnish.

Recipe:

Preheat the oven as per cauliflower crust instructions.

Spread a thin layer of gluten-free tomato sauce over the crust.

Add slices of fresh mozzarella evenly on top.

Pizza should be baked until the cheese has melted and the crust is golden.

Take out of the oven and add some fresh basil leaves on top.

Drizzle with extra virgin olive oil before slicing and serving.

These recipes are not only delicious but also gluten-free, ensuring that those with dietary restrictions can enjoy flavorful and satisfying dinners. Each recipe comes with pre-tips to guide novices through the cooking process seamlessly. Whether you're a beginner or an experienced cook, these gluten-free dinner ideas are sure to become favorites in your household.

CHAPTER TEN

GLUTEN-FREE SNACK ATTACK OPTIONS

Wholesome and Delicious Gluten-Free Snacks:

Creating a variety of wholesome and delicious gluten-free snacks is not only a necessity for those with celiac disease but can also be a delightful exploration of flavors and textures. One fantastic option is gluten-free energy bites. These bite-sized wonders are not only easy to make but also packed with nutritious ingredients. To begin, gather gluten-free oats, nut butter, honey, and add-ins like dried fruits or nuts. In a large bowl, combine the oats and nut butter, drizzling in honey for sweetness. Mix in your chosen add-ins, shaping the mixture into small, bite-sized balls. Refrigerate for a few hours to firm them up, and voilà – you have a batch of scrumptious energy bites ready to satisfy your snack cravings.

Another delightful gluten-free snack is homemade popcorn with unique flavor twists. Traditional popcorn is naturally gluten-free, but it's the seasonings that can often pose a challenge. Make a savory batch by drizzling melted butter over the popped corn and sprinkling it with gluten-free nutritional yeast for a cheesy flavor. For a sweet option, toss popcorn with cinnamon and a touch of sugar. Experimenting with different spices allows for a diverse range of gluten-free popcorn options, providing a satisfying crunch for any snacking occasion.

Dive into the world of gluten-free granola bars to add a nutritious and portable snack to your repertoire. Begin by combining gluten-free oats, nuts, seeds, and dried fruits in a bowl. In a saucepan, heat honey and nut butter until well combined, then pour the mixture over the dry ingredients. Press the mixture into a lined pan, refrigerate until set, and cut into bars. These gluten-free granola bars not only make for a convenient snack but also allow for endless customization, tailoring the ingredients to suit personal preferences and dietary needs.

Techniques for Reducing Gluten in Snacking:

For those navigating a gluten-free lifestyle, it's crucial to become adept at identifying and mitigating gluten content in snacks. One effective technique is to opt for naturally gluten-free whole foods. Fresh fruits, vegetables, cheeses, and nuts are excellent choices, ensuring that you enjoy a satisfying snack without the worry of hidden gluten. Pairing apple slices with almond butter or enjoying a handful of mixed nuts can provide a nutrient-rich and gluten-free snack experience.

Reading labels with diligence is a fundamental skill in reducing gluten intake. Food manufacturers are required to list potential allergens, including wheat, on product labels. Learn to recognize gluten-containing ingredients such as wheat, barley, and rye. Additionally, be cautious of hidden gluten in additives like modified food starch or malt flavoring. Familiarizing oneself with safe and unsafe ingredients empowers individuals to make informed choices, minimizing the risk of accidental gluten consumption.

Embrace the art of substitution when transforming favorite snacks into gluten-free alternatives. Gluten-free flour, such as almond, coconut, or rice flour, can replace traditional wheat flour in recipes. Experimenting with these alternatives allows for the creation of gluten-free versions of muffins, cookies, and other baked treats. Utilize gluten-free breadcrumbs for coating or as a topping to maintain the crunch in favorite recipes. By becoming comfortable with substitution, individuals can continue to enjoy their favorite snacks without compromising on taste or texture.

In conclusion, mastering the creation of wholesome gluten-free snacks and implementing techniques for reducing gluten in snacking can open up a world of delicious possibilities for those following a celiac disease diet. Whether it's crafting energy bites, exploring unique popcorn flavors, or perfecting gluten-free granola bars, the key lies in creativity, label literacy, and the willingness to embrace alternative ingredients. With these skills in hand, even novices can confidently navigate the realm of gluten-free snacking, savoring every bite without the worry of gluten-induced discomfort.

More Additional Gluten-Free Snacks Ideas And Pre Tips

Gluten-Free Snack Idea 1: Quinoa-Stuffed Bell Peppers:

Take a savory turn with these gluten-free quinoa-stuffed bell peppers, providing a satisfying and nutritious snack option. Begin by cooking the quinoa according to the package instructions. In a pan, sauté a mix of vegetables like diced tomatoes, onions, and spinach. Combine the cooked quinoa with the sautéed vegetables, adding herbs and spices for flavor. Cut bell peppers in half, remove seeds, and stuff them with the quinoa mixture. Bake until the peppers are tender. This gluten-free snack not only satisfies cravings but also offers a boost of protein and fiber, making it a wholesome choice for any time of the day.

Pre-Tip: When choosing quinoa, ensure it's labeled gluten-free, as cross-contamination can occur during processing. Rinse the quinoa thoroughly before cooking to remove any residue that may contain traces of gluten.

Gluten-Free Snack Idea 2: Rice Paper Spring Rolls:

Explore the refreshing world of gluten-free rice paper spring rolls, a versatile snack that allows for endless customization. Soak rice paper sheets in warm water until pliable, then lay them on a flat surface. Fill the center with a combination of gluten-free ingredients such as shrimp, rice noodles, fresh herbs, and crisp vegetables. Fold the sides over the filling and roll tightly. These spring rolls can be served with a gluten-free dipping sauce, adding a delightful crunch and burst of flavors to your snack repertoire.

Pre-Tip: Check the labels of rice paper and dipping sauces to ensure they are free from gluten. Use a separate, clean surface to assemble each roll to prevent cross-contamination.

Gluten-Free Snack Idea 3: Yogurt Parfait with Gluten-Free Granola:

Indulge in a sweet and satisfying gluten-free snack by creating a yogurt parfait with gluten-free granola. Choose a yogurt labeled gluten-free or opt for dairy-free alternatives like coconut or almond yogurt. Layer the yogurt with fresh berries and a generous sprinkle of gluten-free granola. This snack not only provides a delightful combination of textures and flavors but also offers a dose of probiotics from the yogurt and essential nutrients from the fruit and granola.

Pre-Tip: Carefully read the labels of both yogurt and granola to ensure they are free from gluten and any potential contaminants. Choose plain yogurt to control the added sugars, and consider making your gluten-free granola at home for complete ingredient control.

Incorporating these additional gluten-free snack ideas into your repertoire, along with the provided pre-tips, ensures a delicious and safe snacking experience. Whether you're in the mood for a savory quinoa-stuffed bell pepper, a refreshing rice paper spring roll, or a sweet yogurt parfait, these recipes cater to a variety of tastes while keeping gluten concerns at bay.

CHAPTER ELEVEN

RICH, GLUTEN-FREE SWEET TREATS

Recipes For Decadent Desserts Without Gluten:

Embracing the rich tapestry of flavors and textures achievable with substitute flours and ingredients is crucial when venturing into the world of exquisite gluten-free desserts. The delicious flourless chocolate cake is one such instance. High-quality dark chocolate, butter, eggs, and sugar are the key ingredients in this delicious dessert, which is naturally gluten-free velvety, and rich. The taste and satisfaction are unaffected by the lack of typical flour; in fact, the chocolatey experience is enhanced beyond recognition.

The gluten-free berry tart is a tasty alternative for everyone who enjoys fruity sweetness. Start with a buttery gluten-free crust, which is often produced for the ideal texture using a combination of rice flour, almond flour, and xanthan gum. Strawberries, blueberries, and raspberries combine to form a mélange and fill this golden crust, adding a pop of color and natural flavor. This tart's glossy sheen comes from a simple glaze made with gluten-free apricot preserves, which elevates it from a delicious dessert to a work of art.

Make a new version of the classic brownie by using gluten-free ingredients. To get a fudgy and moist texture, use a blend of almond flour and coconut flour in place of regular wheat flour. For an extra-indulgent touch, add a good handful of gluten-free chocolate chips and premium cocoa powder. These brownies demonstrate that sweets free of gluten may be just as decadent and filling as traditional desserts.

Experimentation is the secret to gluten-free decadence. Explore the world of alternative flours such as buckwheat flour, chickpea flour, and sorghum flour to find new flavors and textures to add to your repertoire of gluten-free desserts. The secret is to embrace the diversity of products devoid of gluten and let your imagination run wild.

Baking Hints for Sweet Treats Without Gluten:

Taking up gluten-free baking demands a mental adjustment as well as a thorough knowledge of substitute components. Purchasing premium gluten-free flour is the first step toward getting the right flavor and texture. The greatest results are frequently obtained from blends that include a range of flours, including tapioca, almond, and rice flour. Moreover, adding xanthan gum can replicate the gluten's binding qualities, giving your baked goods structure.

Precise measurements are essential for successful gluten-free baking. For a more accurate and reliable result, use measuring cups made especially for gluten-free flour. Weighing ingredients is also helpful since it guarantees a precise balance and lowers the possibility of an excessively dense or dry finished product.

It's liberating to know the science behind baking without gluten. Different types of flour give your recipes unique features.

Coconut flour delivers lightness and absorbency, while almond flour adds moisture and richness. By experimenting with different flour mixtures, you can customize your recipes to your liking.

Ingredients must be used at room temperature for best results. Let the butter, eggs, and dairy substitutes come to room temperature before adding them to your batter. This guarantees adequate emulsification and a more uniform dispersion of components, culminating in a more velvety and appetizing consistency.

When it comes to baking gluten-free, patience is key. Before baking, give your dough or batter a few minutes to rest. This improves the texture overall and keeps the mouthfeel from being grainy by allowing the flours to fully hydrate. Accept the process of learning by doing, keeping in mind that every oven and gluten-free flour blend will react differently.

In summary, baking without gluten presents a chance for gastronomic experimentation rather than a restriction.

If you have the correct information and are prepared to try new things, even beginners can make incredibly rich and tasty gluten-free desserts that are on par with their gluten-containing counterparts.

CHAPTER TWELVE

CREATING A BALANCED GLUTEN-FREE MEAL PLAN
A Comprehensive Guide for Organizing Gluten-Free Meals:

For those with celiac disease, especially those who are new to the diet, meal planning may initially seem challenging. However, if you dissect it into manageable steps, it may become less daunting and more of a simple process.

1. **Understanding the Basics of Eating Gluten-Free:** It's critical to understand which foods are inherently gluten-free and which are not. Typical gluten-containing foods include rye, barley, and wheat; gluten-free foods include rice, quinoa, and maize. Find information about gluten-free cereals, fruits, vegetables, dairy products, and proteins.

2. **Create a Gluten-Free Pantry:** Creating a gluten-free haven in your kitchen is crucial and

should be your top priority. Purchase gluten-free flour blends instead of regular flour, and make sure you have an ample supply of pasta, rice, and quinoa that are free of gluten. Separate toasters, cutting boards, and utensils that are solely supposed to be used for gluten-free cooking to prevent cross-contamination in your pantry.

3. Accept Whole Foods: The foundation of a well-balanced gluten-free diet plan is whole, naturally gluten-free foods. Options for lean protein include fish, poultry, and legumes. Stuff your plate with colorful fruits and vegetables to ensure that it is nutrient-dense. Whole foods add greater variation to your meals in addition to improving nutrition.

4. Create Weekly Menus: When you plan your meals, knowing what to eat each day doesn't have to be difficult. Make a weekly menu with a range of gluten-free fruits, vegetables, meats, and grains. This will lessen the likelihood that you may stray from your gluten-free diet when supermarket shopping.

5. Examine Various Gluten-Free Recipes: Try some gluten-free recipes to give your meals a unique touch. There are countless delicious selections to satisfy a wide range of preferences. Try experimenting with new cooking methods and taste combinations to keep your meals interesting. Online, there are a plethora of gluten-free recipes to fit any type of culinary style.

6. Practice Mindful Eating and amount management: In addition to gluten-free foods, it's important to stress mindful eating and amount management. Placing the appropriate amounts of proteins, carbohydrates, and fats on your plate will guarantee a well-rounded lunch. Learn to trust your body's hunger and fullness cues to help you develop a healthy relationship with food.

Balancing Variety and Nutrition:

To meet your body's needs and enjoy a broad variety of flavors, a well-balanced gluten-free meal plan considers both variety and nutrition.

1. Nutrient-rich foods: To ensure that you're getting enough vitamins and minerals, choose foods that are high in nutrients. Include gluten-free whole grains, lean meats, and an array of vibrantly colored fruits and vegetables. These choices not only provide necessary nutrients but also contribute to a satisfying and well-rounded dinner.

2. Protein Power: A well-balanced diet has to contain some protein. Include a variety of protein sources, such as tofu, fish, eggs, lentils, and fowl. This variety not only meets your protein needs but also adds more taste and texture to your meals. To make your protein choices interesting, experiment with different cooking methods.

3. Nutritious Fats: Feel free to incorporate nuts and other healthy fats into your gluten-free diet. Extra virgin olive oil, avocados, nuts, and seeds are excellent providers of essential fatty acids. These fats improve the taste of your food and also aid in fullness and general health.

4. Mix Up Your Grains: While eliminating grains that contain gluten, increase the variety of grains you eat that are gluten-free. Try different combinations of quinoa, brown rice, millet, and buckwheat to make sure the flavors and textures are varied. This gives you a wider range of nutrients and also adds diversity to your diet.

5. Keep an Eye on the Micronutrients: Make sure the gluten-free meal plan includes all the important micronutrients. To ensure a variety of vitamins and minerals, including a choice of fruits and vegetables. To provide your body with a variety of nutrients and enhance your general health, think about switching up your choices once a week.

6. Hydration and Dietary Fiber: Two sometimes missed but essential components of a well-balanced gluten-free diet are adequate hydration and dietary fiber. Fiber promotes gut health, and water aids in digestion and nutritional absorption. To maintain maximum health, include lots of foods high in water and gluten-free sources of fiber, such as fruits, vegetables, and whole grains.

Therefore, creating a well-balanced diet by adding a variety of nutrient-rich foods into meal planning requires a methodical approach.

Enjoying entire foods, experimenting with recipes, and paying attention to portion sizes all help make eating gluten-free gratifying and pleasurable. Maintaining a healthy, tasty, and long-lasting gluten-free diet requires striking a balance between variety and nutrition.

CHAPTER THIRTEEN

HANDLING SOCIAL CIRCUMSTANCES AND EATING OUT

Advice For People With Celiac Disease

For those with celiac disease, navigating restaurants and eating out might be difficult, but it is completely manageable with the correct strategy and understanding. Finding eateries that provide gluten-free food is the first step for a novice. Locate businesses that prioritize gluten-free practices by using online resources, such as websites and apps for gluten-free restaurants. Customer evaluations can offer important information about a restaurant's commitment to serving gluten-free food, so pay attention to them.

It's important to phone the restaurant you've selected in advance to let them know about any dietary requirements you may have. By taking this proactive measure, you enable the restaurant personnel to get ready for your visit and guarantee a more seamless dining experience. Make sure the staff members understand how serious your disease is and how crucial it is to prevent cross-contamination.

Ask inquiries regarding the menu and preparation techniques as soon as you arrive at the restaurant. If a gluten-free menu is offered, ask to see it. You should also ask about ingredients and possible cross-contamination hazards. Reputable eateries will recognize your efforts to ensure a safe dinner because they are used to accommodating special dietary requirements.

Be explicit about your need for a gluten-free meal when placing your order. Make it very clear that there are no gluten-containing components or cross-contamination hazards in the food you make. To reduce the possibility of concealed gluten, choose straightforward recipes made with raw, naturally gluten-free products. Salads, grilled veggies, and meats are frequently healthy options.

You still need to be on the lookout after placing your order. Remind your server politely of your requirement for a gluten-free meal and stress how serious cross-contamination is. To prevent any misunderstandings, make sure the kitchen crew is informed of your dietary needs. Never be afraid to ask to speak with the chef directly if you have any questions or concerns.

It's also a good idea to be prepared with gluten-free snacks, particularly if you're eating somewhere with few gluten-free options. In the unlikely event that the restaurant is unable to sufficiently meet your demands, having a little food on hand guarantees that you won't go hungry. Furthermore, retaining an optimistic and forgiving demeanor during the meal can facilitate a more cooperative and empathetic exchange with the restaurant personnel.

In summary, eating out with having celiac disease necessitates careful planning, prompt communication, and a sharp understanding of the hazards. You may have a wonderful and safe gluten-free lunch by choosing places that are celiac-friendly, making sure you communicate your needs properly, and being watchful during the entire eating experience.

Managing Social Events and Get-togethers while Following a Gluten-Free Diet:

Social activities and get-togethers can present particular difficulties for people with celiac disease, but these circumstances can be effectively managed with careful preparation and communication. The secret for a beginner is to take charge of your food requirements and still enjoy the social parts of activities.

Notifying the event organizers in advance of your dietary limitations is one useful tactic. Tell the host about your gluten-free needs whether it's a corporate function, a wedding, or a family get-together. By informing them in advance, the host can make modifications and guarantees that you will have appropriate choices.

If you're not sure what's on the menu at a social gathering, think about bringing something gluten-free to share. This not only ensures that you'll have a safe meal alternative, but it also teaches people how to cook without gluten. From appetizers to desserts, there are a plethora of delectable gluten-free dishes that can suit a variety of palates.

When you go to a potluck or buffet-style gathering, be cautious when handling the food spread. Ask the host for details on the dishes or take the initiative to find out about the ingredients. To reduce the possibility of unintentional gluten exposure, use separate serving utensils and refrain from sharing condiments. Keep in mind that cross-contamination is a potential concern.

If you are hosting an event that is catered or at a business luncheon where you have little influence over the menu, quietly discuss your dietary requirements with the caterer or event organizers. The majority of catering firms can offer advice on safe food selections and are experienced in meeting different dietary requirements.

When expressing your demands to others regarding gluten avoidance, it's critical to be both assertive and courteous. Inform your coworkers, acquaintances, and family about the existence of gluten-containing components and the symptoms of celiac disease. Thanking them for their cooperation and understanding helps build a supportive environment and increase knowledge about living a gluten-free lifestyle.

In conclusion, proactive communication, preparation, and a desire to teach others are essential for handling social gatherings and events with celiac disease. It is possible to enjoy social events and prioritize your health at the same time by being upfront about your dietary requirements, offering to provide gluten-free meals, and using caution when handling food spreads.

FINAL THOUGHT

Summary of Main Ideas:

Before beginning a gluten-free journey, it is important to review and make sense of the main ideas presented in the "Celiac Disease Diet Cookbook." A thorough awareness of the dietary limitations brought on by celiac disease is the cornerstone of healthy gluten-free living. Start by going over the fundamental ideas that set gluten-free and gluten-containing meals apart. This entails closely examining gluten-containing foods including wheat, barley, and rye as well as paying close attention to ingredient labels. Stress the value of being cautious and avoiding cross-contamination when dining at restaurants.

After you have a good handle on the fundamentals, explore the range of substitute grains and flours that can easily take the place of their gluten-containing equivalents. Describe the differences between grains that are gluten-free, such as quinoa, rice, and maize, and offer helpful hints for incorporating them into regular meals. Making grocery shopping easier for newcomers can be achieved by offering a list of staple gluten-free products along with suggested brands. Stress the need to create a nutrient-dense, well-rounded diet to make up for any possible nutrient shortages brought on by cutting out gluten-containing cereals.

Moving on to the kitchen, investigate the methods that maximize cooking that is free of gluten. Teach beginners the basics of baking without gluten by offering dependable recipes for cakes, cookies, and bread. Emphasize how important it is to use gluten alternatives like tapioca flour and xanthan gum to get the right texture and consistency. Provide examples of meal planning techniques that not only make cooking gluten-free easier to handle but also more pleasurable. A methodical approach to cooking gluten-free food can boost beginners' confidence and make the kitchen a comfortable place for them to work.

Motivation and Support for Sustaining a Happy, Gluten-Free Lifestyle:

Success in maintaining a gluten-free lifestyle demands more than just following dietary recommendations; it also calls for a resilient mindset and persistent motivation. Encourage people to start this path by emphasizing the positive changes that a gluten-free diet may bring about in terms of general health and wellbeing. Tell success stories of people who have overcome the obstacles posed by celiac disease to demonstrate that a rich and meaningful life is achievable with commitment and knowledge.

Shared experiences and a feeling of community are typically the sources of motivation. Urge newcomers to join online and offline support groups to help them feel like they belong and to provide them with a place to discuss strategies and difficulties. Recognize that there may occasionally be challenges and failures, but stress the perseverance required to get past them. Discuss the long-term advantages of living a gluten-free lifestyle, including how it can help manage celiac disease and enhance general health and vigor.

Include techniques for motivating people, such as making realistic goals and acknowledging little accomplishments along the way. Remind newcomers that as their comfort with a gluten-free lifestyle increases, the first difficulties will disappear. Provide advice on how to stick to a gluten-free diet when traveling, eating out, and navigating social situations. Through the cultivation of an optimistic and self-sufficient mindset, beginners can confidently embark on their gluten-free path, setting the stage for long-term success and good health.

MY GRATITUDES

Dear Valued Readers and Supporters,

I hope this message finds you well. I am writing to express my deepest gratitude to both God and each one of you for the overwhelming support and positive response to my book. Your encouragement and enthusiasm have truly touched my heart, and I am immensely thankful for the journey we are on together.

I believe that every success is a result of collaboration and support from various sources. First and foremost, I want to acknowledge the divine guidance and inspiration that led me to create this cookbook. Without the grace of God, this endeavor would not have been possible.

To my cherished readers, your commitment to exploring healthier dietary options for managing your crises has been both inspiring and humbling. Your trust in this book" means the world to me, and I am honored to be part of your journey toward improved health and well-being.

Also, I am reaching out to kindly request your valuable feedback on this book. Your thoughts and insights are crucial in helping me enhance and serve you better, ensuring that it continues to meet your needs effectively. Please take a moment to share your thoughts by rating and writing reviews on platforms where the book is available.

Your reviews not only provide me with invaluable feedback but also play a significant role in assisting others in making informed choices. By sharing your experiences, you contribute to a community that values health and wellness, creating a positive impact on countless lives.

Additionally, I encourage you to share this book with your friends, family and loved ones.

Together, we can extend the reach of this promising resource, offering support and guidance to those who may benefit from it. Having this knowledge and seeking medical advice from your specialist I anticipate a turnaround for us.

Once again, thank you from the depths of my heart for your unwavering support. I am committed to continually improving and serving you better. Let us continue this journey together, promoting health, well-being, and a shared sense of community.

With sincere appreciation,

[Emmy Brooks]

Author, "CELIAC DISEASE DIET COOKBOOK"